The Intrinsic Core

using the soft gym overball

© 2006 Caroline Corning Creager

The Intrinsic Core
using the soft gym overball

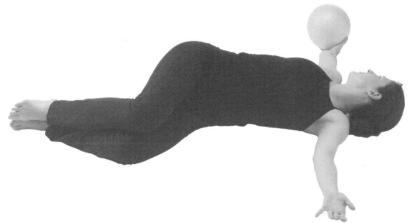

© 2006 Caroline Corning Creager

www.carolinecreager.com

Published by:

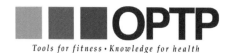

Tools for fitness · Knowledge for health

Creager, Caroline Corning
    The Intrinsic Core: using the soft gym overball
    Creager, Caroline Corning - 1st edition

For information contact:

OPTP
3800 Annapolis Lane Suite 165
Minneapolis, MN 55447
(800) 367-7393
www.optp.com

The author has made every effort to assure that the information in this book is accurate and current at the time of printing. The publisher and author take no responsibility for the use of the material in this book and cannot be held responsible for any typographical or other errors found. Please consult your physician before initiating this exercise program. The information in this book is not intended to replace medical advice.

ISBN: 0 - 9771378 - 6 - 4; 978 - 0 - 9771378 - 6 - 2

Cover Design by Jeff Polley
Book Design by Jeff Polley
Photographs by NEXT Communications/Terry Anderson Photography

Printed in the United States of America

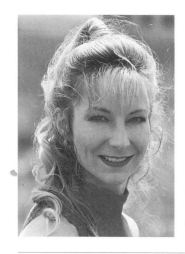

About the Author:

Caroline Corning Creager, P.T.

Caroline Corning Creager is an award-winning author and an internationally recognized speaker on fitness and physical therapy topics. Caroline received her degree in Physical Therapy from the University of Montana. She is the Owner and C.E.O. of FitNiche Publishing, the Berthoud Athletic Club, and Executive Physical Therapy, Inc. in Berthoud, Colorado, U.S.A., and author of eight books: *Bounce Back Into Shape After Baby, Therapeutic Exercises Using Foam Rollers, Therapeutic Exercises Using the Swiss Ball, Therapeutic Exercises Using Resistive Bands, Caroline Creager's Airobic Ball Strengthening Workout, Caroline Creager's Airobic Ball Stretching Workout, Core Strength Training Using Inflatable and Foam Rollers,* and *The Intrinsic Core: using the soft gym overball.*

She has written or been featured in numerous national and international magazines: *Cooking Light, Fitness, Fit, Tennis, Yoga Journal, Massage Journal, WorldWideSpine, PhysioForum, Advance for PT's, Advance for OT's, Advance for Nurses, Idea Personal Trainer,* and *Baby Steps,* and has been a guest speaker on local and national television programs including *America's Talking: Alive and Wellness,* and the *Rehab Training Network.*

Table of Contents

Introduction..1

BASIC CORE EXERCISES 2

Scapular Stabilizer 3
Transverse Abdominis Exercise 4
Kegel 5
Hip Stabilizer with Transverse Abdominis Exercise........6

STRETCHES 7

Shoulder Stretch...8
Chest Stretch..9
Pelvic Tilts 10
Sidelying Spinal Twist...11
Sidelying Quadricep Stretch 12
Hamstring Stretch...13
Hip Stretch..14
Buttock Stretch 15
Lower Back Stretch 16

STRENGTHENING EXERCISES 17

Rotator Cuff Rotation...18
Prone Row and Press 19
Side Bridge with Rotation of Rotator Cuff.....................20
Hip Raise and Roll...21
Hip Raise with Hand Press..22
Knee Lifts 23
Half Locust 24
Back Stabilizer..25
Back Stabilizer with Arm Raise.....................................26
Back Stabilizer with Arm and Leg Raise........................27
Starting Block Abdominal Strengthener.........................28
Abdominal 'V' 29
Oblique Crunch 30
Pelvic Floor Strengthener 31
Hip Twister..32
Thigh Squeeze 33
Hip Stabilizer 34
Bicycle 35
Pilates Leg Raises...36
Straight Leg Raises 37
Standing Heel Slides on Wall 38
Mini-Squat with Ball Between Knees.............................39
Mini-Squat with Shoulder Press Into Wall 40
Mini-Squat with Shoulder Protraction/Retraction..........41
Mini-Squat with Tricep Extension 42
Mini-Squat with Arm Raises 43
Modified Cactus Pose 44

References 45

Introduction

The Soft Gym Overball: A well-rounded core strengthener

For a well-rounded fitness tool to support your core strengthening exercise routine, there's nothing simpler than the Soft Gym Overball. Sometimes referred to as a Pilates ball, the Soft Gym Overball is a small, burst-resistant globe that helps you focus your core muscle exercises, add resistance to movements, and improve your overall balance.

The core muscles—abdominals to back and hips, pelvic floor to diaphragm—provide the infrastructure for every movement of the body. Using the Soft Gym Overball to enhance the core-strengthening benefits of your fitness regimen can promote better overall results in every area of the body you want to tone. For defined abdominals, a stronger upper body, and toned arms and legs, the exercises included in this book begin with strengthening the core muscles and the results will radiate outward.

About the Soft Gym Overball

The Soft Gym Overball ball is lightweight, compact and easy to use. At 23 cm. in diameter, it is extremely portable and can be inflated on-the-fly. One of the few air-filled fitness tools than can be inflated by mouth, the ball comes with a straw so you can blow it up with just a few puffs, or use a hand or foot pump. It also deflates quickly and easily so it is convenient for travel.

Do I need a special ball to perform these exercises?

Unlike a child's toy or a sports ball, the Soft Gym Overball is designed to support the pressure applied during specific exercises. Made of burst-resistant pvc foam, the Soft Gym Overball can support 400 pounds of pressure. The ball's surface is smooth and non-irritating so that you can comfortably press against it. It is safe for individuals with sensitivity to latex.

How do I clean my ball?

For home use, clean the Soft Gym Overball with soap and water. In the clinic, use a mild disinfectant such as you would use on any vinyl surface.

What exercises should I do first?

It is important to establish a basic level of fitness in the core muscles before proceeding to any of the fitness ball exercises in this book. The muscle groups of the core—the diaphragm, abdominal, back, hip and pelvic floor muscles—play an essential role in supporting the pelvis, spine and abdomen. As the fitness ball exercises each require an understanding of how to stabilize your core, you must first make sure that you can locate these muscle groups and learn to engage them to support the spine.

What do the stars signify on each exercise page?

Each exercise is rated on a one to five star system. One star signifies the most basic exercise level, two stars – advanced beginner, three stars – intermediate, four stars – advanced, and five stars – expert. If the exercise received one star, then you will know that it may be performed by a beginner, and a five star exercise means you may need to wait awhile before you perform it, or that this exercise is for you if you are already in great shape.

BASIC CORE
EXERCISES

Scapular Stabilizer 3

Transverse Abdominis Exercise 4

Kegel 5

Hip Stabilizer with Transverse Abdominis Exercise.....................6

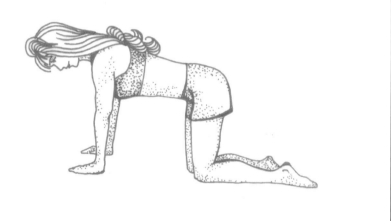

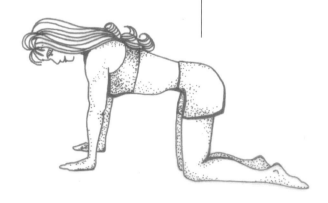

Scapular Stabilizer

Level of Difficulty: ★☆☆☆☆

Benefits: Strengthens mid-back muscles.

HOLD: 5 – 20 seconds

REPEAT: 2 – 10 times

FREQUENCY: 2 – 3 times per day

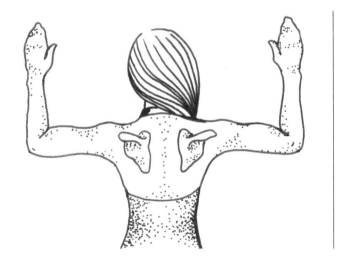 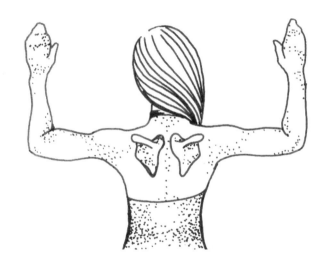

Instructions:

Lie on abdomen with head placed on a small towel roll. Place hands on floor at a 90-degree angle (or less) from body. Relax shoulders and neck. Take a relaxed breath in and out. Now without breathing in, slowly and gently draw the lower abdomen in towards the spine and the shoulder blades down and in—as if squeezing the shoulder blades together. Hold, breathe lightly. Relax the abdomen and shoulder blades.

Transverse Abdominis Exercise

Level of Difficulty: ★☆☆☆☆

Benefits: Strengthens deep abdominal muscles located on side and front of abdomen.

HOLD: 4 – 20 seconds

REPEAT: 5 – 10 times

FREQUENCY: 2 – 3 times per day

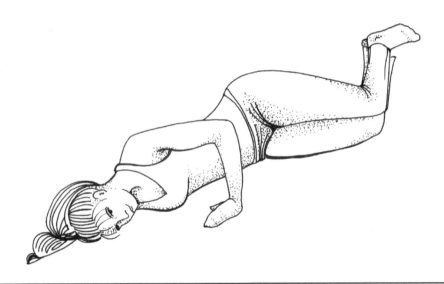

Instructions:
Lie on side with knees bent at a 90-degree angle. Take a relaxed breath in and out. Now without breathing in, slowly and gently draw the lower abdomen in towards the spine. Hold, breathe lightly. Relax the abdomen gradually.

Variation:
This exercise may be performed lying on your abdomen, back, standing and later in sitting.

Kegel

Level of Difficulty: ★ ☆ ☆ ☆ ☆

Benefits: Strengthens pelvic floor muscles.

HOLD: 3 seconds with gradual increase to 20 seconds

REPEAT: 3 – 10 times

FREQUENCY: 3 times per day

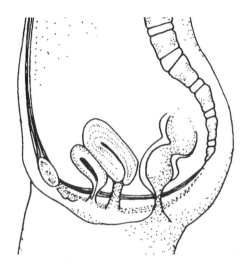 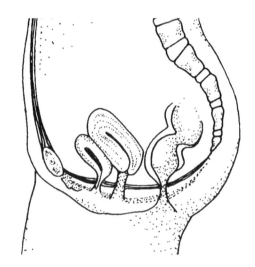

Instructions:
Lie down on back with knees bent and feet shoulder-width apart. Take a relaxed breath in and out. Now without breathing in, slowly draw the pelvic floor muscles up and in as if you are attempting to stop urine flow—keeping buttocks and inner thigh muscles relaxed. Inhale. *Hold* this position for 3 seconds. Gradually relax the pelvic floor muscles for 6 seconds. Once you have mastered this exercise, progress to doing the exercise sitting, standing, or squatting.

Note:
Relaxation period should be twice as long as hold time, until you reach a 10 second hold.

Hip Stabilizer with Transverse Abdominis Exercise

Level of Difficulty: ★☆☆☆☆

Benefits: Strengthens hip and abdominal muscles.

HOLD: 3 seconds

REPEAT: 3 – 10 times

FREQUENCY: 2 – 3 times per day

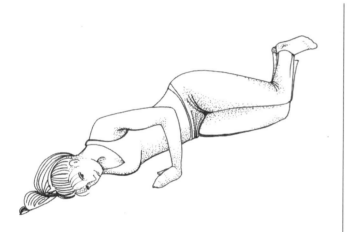
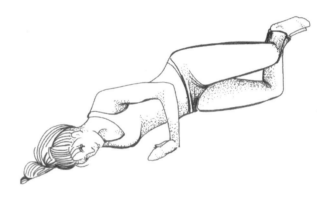

Instructions:

Lie on side with knees bent at a 90-degree angle, keeping a straight line between shoulders, hips and ankles. Take a relaxed breath in and out. Now without breathing in, slowly and gently draw the lower abdomen in towards the spine. Keeping heels together raise knees as far as possible without any hip movement. Lower knees. Repeat on opposite side.

STRETCHES

Shoulder Stretch...8

Chest Stretch...9

Pelvic Tilts 10

Spinal Twist 11

Quadricep Stretch 12

Hamstring Stretch..13

Hip Stretch..14

Buttock Stretch 15

Lower Back Stretch 16

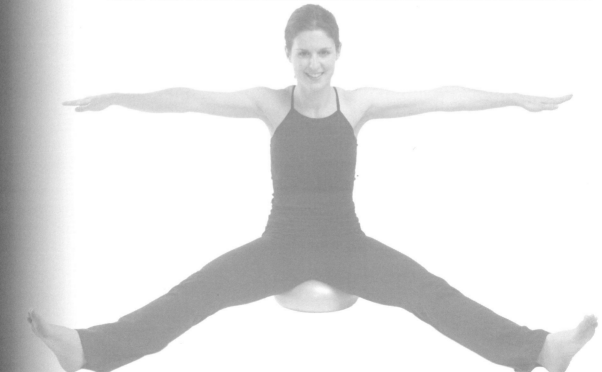

Shoulder Stretch

Level of Difficulty: ★☆☆☆☆

Benefits: Stretches shoulder muscles.

HOLD: 20 seconds

REPEAT: 1 – 3 times

FREQUENCY: daily

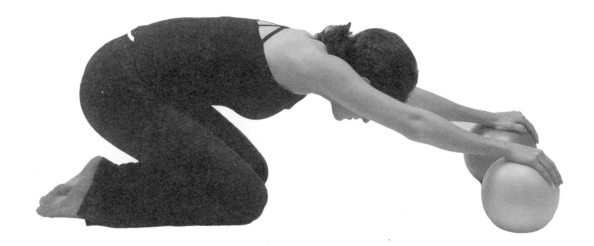

Instructions:
Kneel. Grasp one ball in each hand. Lean forward and place balls on floor. Lower head until you feel a comfortable stretch or ears are lowered between straight arms.

Chest Stretch

Level of Difficulty: ★☆☆☆☆

Benefits: Stretches chest and shoulder muscles.

HOLD: 20 seconds

REPEAT: 1 – 3 times

FREQUENCY: daily

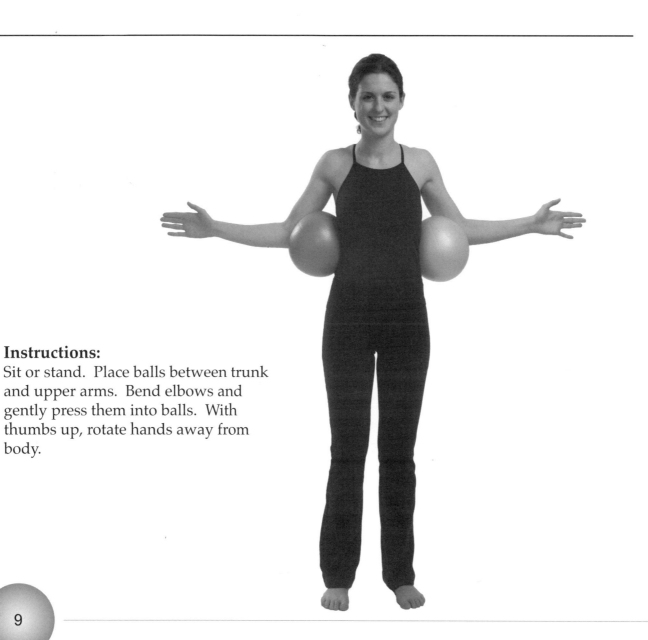

Instructions:
Sit or stand. Place balls between trunk and upper arms. Bend elbows and gently press them into balls. With thumbs up, rotate hands away from body.

Pelvic Tilts

Level of Difficulty: ★ ★ ☆ ☆ ☆

Benefits: Stretches abdomen and back muscles.

HOLD: 5 seconds

REPEAT: 1 – 3 times

FREQUENCY: daily

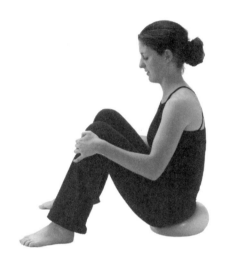 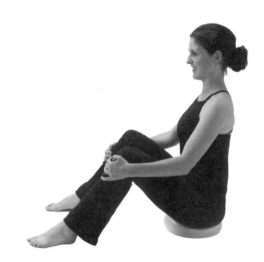

Instructions:
Sit on ball with feet hip-width apart and place hands on knees. Draw lower abdomen toward spine. Roll ball forward as hips roll backward (round back). Return to starting position. Roll ball backward as hips roll forward (arched back). Return to starting position.

Sidelying Spinal Twist

Level of Difficulty: ★☆☆☆☆

Benefits: Stretches trunk and neck muscles.

HOLD: 20 seconds

REPEAT: 1 – 3 times per side

FREQUENCY: daily

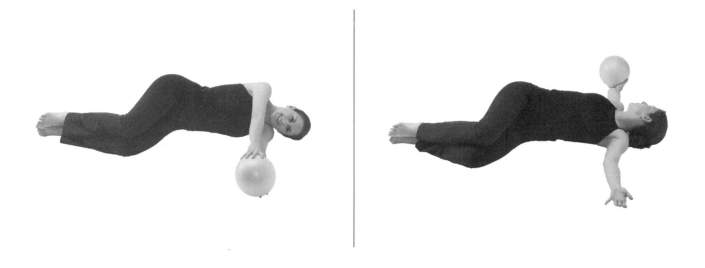

Instructions:
Lie on side and bend knees. Grasp ball lightly in right hand and straighten arms. Gently draw lower abdomen toward spine. With eyes on ball, slowly rotate trunk so right hand is touching floor on opposite side of body. Hold. Return to starting position.

Sidelying Quadricep Stretch

Level of Difficulty: ★☆☆☆☆

Benefits: Stretches quadriceps (front thigh muscles).

HOLD: 20 seconds

REPEAT: 1 – 3 times per side

FREQUENCY: daily

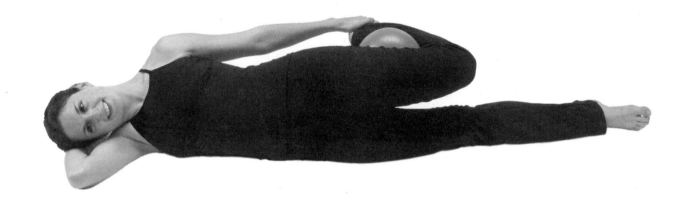

Instructions:
Lie on side. Bend top knee and place ball between calf and thigh. Grasp ankle with hand while maintaining knee alignment with trunk and without arching lower back. Draw heel toward buttock while squeezing ball. Return to starting position. Repeat on opposite side.

Hamstring Stretch

Level of Difficulty: ★☆☆☆☆

Benefits: Stretches the hamstrings (back of thighs) and inner thigh muscles.

HOLD: 20 seconds

REPEAT: 1 – 3 times

FREQUENCY: daily

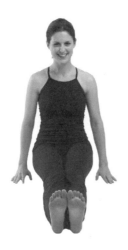 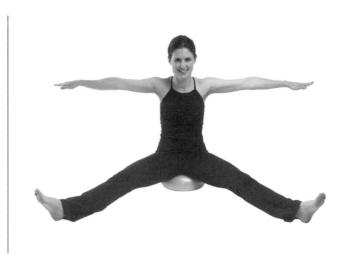

Instructions:
Sit on ball with legs straight out in front of body. Sit up straight and draw lower abdomen toward spine. Flex toes and separate feet as far as comfortable. Raise straight arms out from sides and lean forward until a gentle stretch is felt in the back of thighs.

Hip Stretch

Level of Difficulty: ★ ☆ ☆ ☆ ☆

Benefits: Stretches inner and outer hip muscles.

HOLD: 20 seconds

REPEAT: 1 – 3 times

FREQUENCY: daily

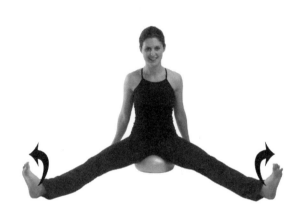 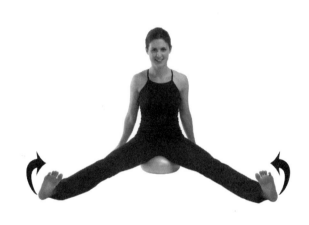

Instructions:
Sit on ball with legs straight and feet as far apart as comfortable. Sit up straight and draw lower abdomen toward spine. Flex toes and rotate feet in and out.

Buttock Stretch

Level of Difficulty: ★☆☆☆☆

Benefits: Stretches buttock muscles.

HOLD: 20 seconds

REPEAT: 1 – 3 times per side

FREQUENCY: daily

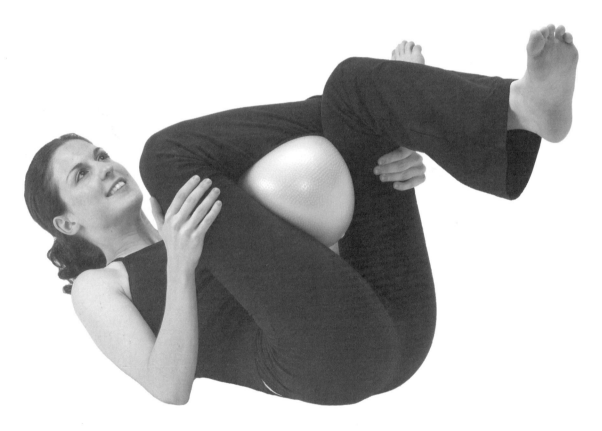

Instructions:
Lie on back with knees bent. Place ball behind right knee and lightly squeeze ball. Rest right ankle across opposite lower thigh. Grasp back of thigh with hands and draw legs to chest until you feel a comfortable stretch. Repeat on opposite side.

Lower Back Stretch

Level of Difficulty: ★☆☆☆☆

Benefits: Stretches lower back and trunk muscles.

HOLD: 20 seconds

REPEAT: 1 – 3 times per side

FREQUENCY: daily

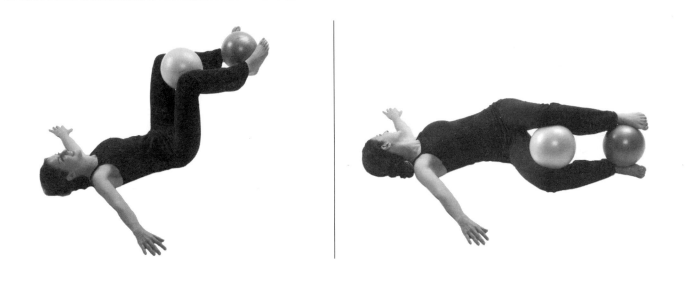

Instructions:
Lie on back with knees bent. Place one ball between knees and one between ankles. Straighten arms out to a "T" position. Gently draw lower abdomen toward spine and knees to chest, keeping knees and hips at 90 degrees. Slowly lower knees to floor or as far as possible without discomfort or arching back.

16

STRENGTHENING EXERCISES

Rotator Cuff Rotation 18

Prone Row and Press 19

Side Bridge with Rotation of Rotator Cuff 20

Hip Raise and Roll 21

Hip Raise with Hand Press 22

Knee Lifts 23

Half Locust 24

Back Stabilizer 25

Back Stabilizer with Arm Raise 26

Back Stabilizer with Arm and Leg Raise 27

Starting Block Abdominal Strengthener 28

Abdominal 'V' 29

Oblique Crunch 30

Pelvic Floor Strengthener 31

Hip Twister 32

Thigh Squeeze 33

Hip Stabilizer 34

Bicycle 35

Pilates Leg Raises 36

Straight Leg Raises 37

Standing Heel Slides on Wall 38

Mini-Squat with Ball Between Knees 39

Mini-Squat with Shoulder Press Into Wall 40

Mini-Squat with Shoulder Protraction/Retraction 41

Mini-Squat with Tricep Extension 42

Mini-Squat with Arm Raises 43

Modified Cactus Pose 44

Rotator Cuff Rotation

Level of Difficulty: ★☆☆☆☆

Benefits: Strengthens rotator cuff muscles.

HOLD: 3 seconds

REPEAT: 8 – 12 times per side

FREQUENCY: daily

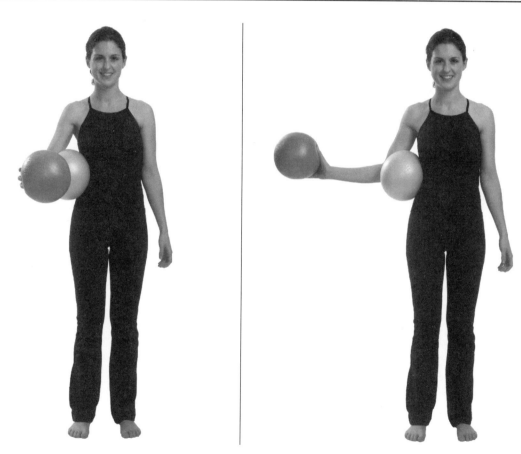

Instructions:
Sit or stand. Place ball between trunk and upper arm and lightly grasp second ball on same side. Bend elbow and gently press it into ball. With thumb up, rotate hand away from body as if pushing a brick wall with the outside of the arm. Return, as if pushing a brick wall with the inside of the arm. Repeat on opposite side.

18

Prone Row and Press

Level of Difficulty: ★ ★ ★ ☆ ☆

Benefits: Strengthens abdomen, chest, back, and mid-back.

HOLD: 3 seconds

REPEAT: 1 – 3 sets, 3 – 8 reps/side

FREQUENCY: 3 – 4 times per week

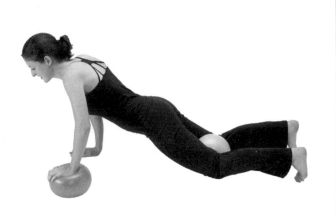 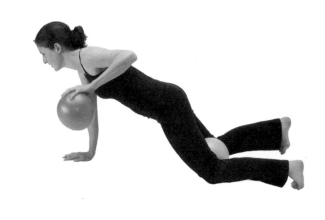

Instructions:
Kneel. Place one ball between knees and one in the palm of your hand. Lean forward so one hand touches floor with palm flat and the other hand presses into ball. Gently draw lower abdomen toward spine. Raise ball off floor and row, keeping shoulder blades down and in. Lower arm and press hand into ball.

Variation:
Perform exercise as above, however raise knees off floor.

Level of Difficulty: ★ ★ ★ ★ ★

Side Bridge with Rotation of Rotator Cuff

Level of Difficulty: ★ ★ ★ ★ ★

Benefits: Strengthens abdomen, back, and rotator cuff muscles.

HOLD: 20 seconds

REPEAT: 3 – 5 times per side

FREQUENCY: daily

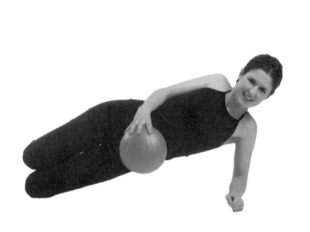 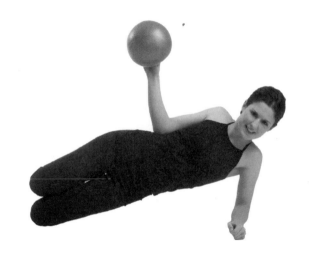

Instructions:
Lie on side and bend knees. Gently draw lower abdomen toward spine. Prop up on left bent elbow so it aligns with shoulder and raise hips off floor. Bend right elbow to 90 degrees and place next to body. Gently grasp ball in right hand and move hand away from body pulling shoulder blades down and in. Return to starting position. Repeat on opposite side.

Hip Raise and Roll

Level of Difficulty: ★☆☆☆☆

Benefits: Strengthens abdominal, buttock, leg and back muscles. Increases space between vertebrae.

HOLD: 1 second for each spinal segment.

REPEAT: 1 – 3 sets, 3 – 6 reps

FREQUENCY: 2 – 3 times per week

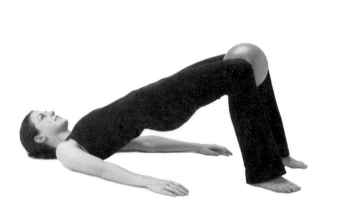 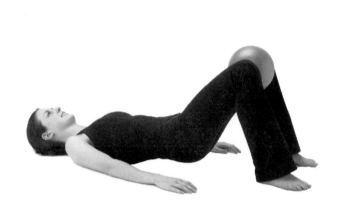

Instructions:

Lie on back with knees bent. Place ball between knees and gently draw lower abdomen toward spine. Raise hips off floor maintaining a line between shoulders, hips and knees. Slowly lower back to floor, one vertebrae at a time, by slowly and gently tilting pelvis posteriorly—as if flattening the back.

Alternate position:

Follow directions above, however after lifting hips off floor—raise arms overhead. Slowly lower back to floor, one vertebrae at a time, by slowly and gently tilting pelvis posteriorly—as if flattening the back.

Hip Raise with Hand Press

Level of Difficulty: ★☆☆☆☆

Benefits: Strengthens buttock, leg and back muscles.

HOLD: 3 seconds

REPEAT: 1 – 3 sets, 8 – 12 reps/side

FREQUENCY: 3 – 4 times per week

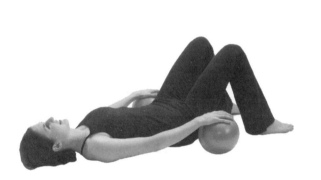 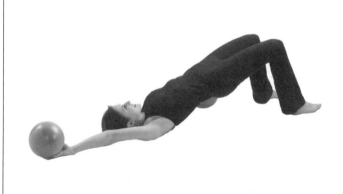

Instructions:
Lie on back with knees bent. Lightly grasp balls in each hand. Gently draw lower abdomen toward spine. Lift hips off floor as you raise right hand overhead and lightly press left hand into ball. Lower hips and arm to floor. Repeat on opposite side.

Knee Lifts

Level of Difficulty: ★ ★ ☆ ☆ ☆

Benefits: Strengthens side abdominal, inner thigh, and neck muscles.

HOLD: 3 seconds

REPEAT: 1 – 3 sets, 6 – 12 reps / side

FREQUENCY: 2 – 3 times per week

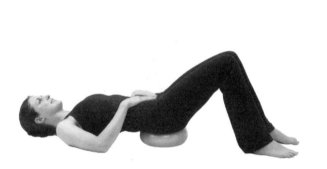 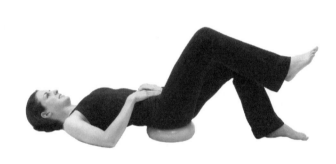

Instructions:
Lie on back with bent knees, hip-width apart. Place ball beneath sacrum (pelvis) and hands on abdomen—monitoring abdominal activity. Gently draw lower abdomen toward spine. Raise right foot off floor. Gently lower foot to floor and repeat on opposite side.

Alternate position:
Follow directions as above, however raise right foot off floor and then raise left foot off floor. Maintain balance with both feet off floor. Repeat exercise by touching right foot to floor and then left.

23

Half Locust

Level of Difficulty: ★ ★ ★ ☆ ☆

Benefits: Strengthens abdomen, back, arms and legs.

HOLD: 3 seconds

REPEAT: 1 – 3 sets, 3 – 8 reps / side

FREQUENCY: 3 – 4 times per week

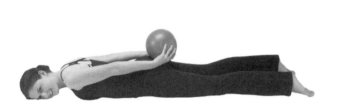
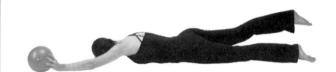

Instructions:
Lie on abdomen. Place hands behind back and ball between palms. Gently draw lower abdomen toward spine. Rotate head to the left and rest cheek on floor. Press hands into ball and release. Grasp ball with left arm and raise overhead as you turn head to the right and lift right leg 3 inches from floor. Return to starting position with hands behind back. Repeat on opposite side.

Note:
If you are unable to place hands behind back, rest them next to the sides of your body.

Back Stabilizer

Level of Difficulty: ★ ★ ★ ☆ ☆

Benefits: Strengthens back, abdomen, arms and leg muscles.

HOLD: 3 seconds

REPEAT: 1 – 3 sets, 8 – 12 reps / side

FREQUENCY: 3 – 4 times per week

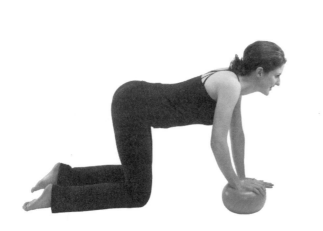 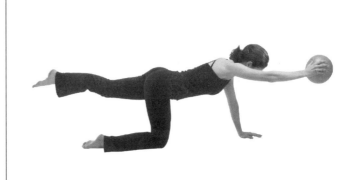

Instructions:
Kneel. Lean forward and place left palm on floor and right palm down on ball—wrists should be in alignment with shoulders. Bend right arm and press palm lightly into ball. Raise right arm straight out in front and opposite leg straight back. Repeat with opposite side.

Variation:
Perform exercise as above, however raise just the arm or just the leg.

Level of Difficulty: ★ ★ ☆ ☆ ☆

Back Stabilizer with Arm Raise

Level of Difficulty: ★ ★ ★ ☆ ☆

Benefits: Strengthens back, abdomen, and arm muscles.

HOLD: 3 seconds

REPEAT: 1– 3 sets, 8 – 12 reps / side

FREQUENCY: 3 – 4 times per week

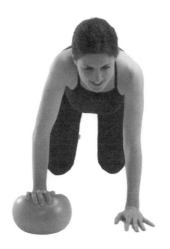 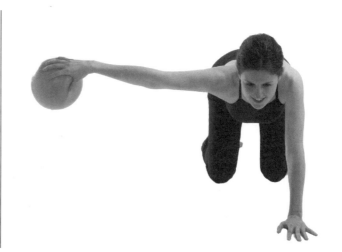

Instructions:

Kneel. Lean forward and place left palm on floor and right palm down on ball—wrists should be in alignment with shoulders. Bend right arm and press palm lightly into ball. Gently draw lower abdomen toward spine and shoulder blades down and in. Raise straight right arm out to the side of body making a 90 degree angle with body. Repeat with opposite side.

Back Stabilizer with Arm and Leg Raise

Level of Difficulty: ★ ★ ★ ★ ★

Benefits: Strengthens back, abdomen, arm and leg muscles.

HOLD: 3 seconds

REPEAT: 1 – 3 sets, 3 – 8 reps / side

FREQUENCY: 3 – 4 times per week

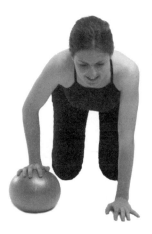 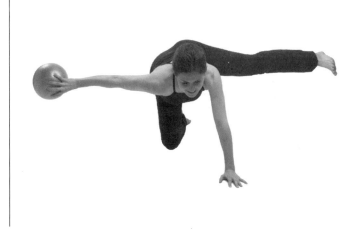

Instructions:
Kneel. Lean forward and place left palm on floor and right palm down on ball—wrists should be in alignment with shoulders. Bend right arm and press palm lightly into ball. Gently draw lower abdomen toward spine and shoulder blades down and in. Raise straight right arm and left leg out to the side of body making 90 degree angles with body. Repeat with opposite side.

Starting Block Abdominal Strengthener

Level of Difficulty: ★ ★ ★ ★ ★

Benefits: Strengthens back, abdomen, arms and legs.

REPEAT: 20 – 60 seconds

FREQUENCY: daily

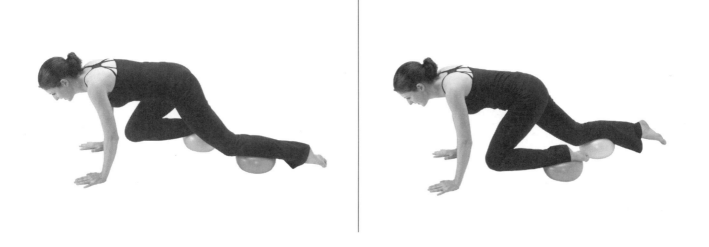

Instructions:
Kneel. Lean forward and place palms on floor—wrists should be in alignment with shoulders. Place a ball under each shin. Gently draw lower abdomen toward spine. Rapidly draw one knee at a time toward the chest, as if running.

Variation:
Perform exercise as above, however slowly draw one knee to chest and return to starting position. Slowly draw opposite knee to chest and return to starting position.

Level of Difficulty: ★ ★ ☆ ☆ ☆

Abdominal 'V'

Level of Difficulty: ★ ★ ★ ★ ★

Benefits: Strengthens side abdominal, inner thigh, and neck muscles.

HOLD: 3 seconds

REPEAT: 1 – 3 sets, 3 – 8 reps

FREQUENCY: 2 – 3 times per week

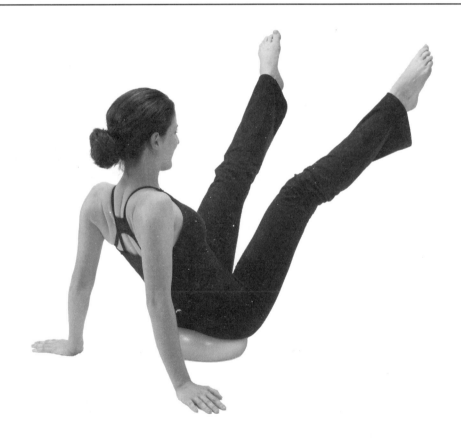

Instructions:
Sit on floor with knees bent. Recline back with bent elbows, aligning elbows underneath shoulders and ball beneath sacrum (pelvis). Gently squeeze shoulder blades together and draw lower abdomen toward spine. Raise both feet off floor, one bent knee at a time. Slowly straighten legs and point toes. Hold. Bend knees and return to starting position.

Oblique Crunch

Level of Difficulty: ★ ★ ★ ☆ ☆

Benefits: Strengthens side abdominal, inner thigh, and neck muscles.

HOLD: 2 seconds

REPEAT: 1 – 3 sets, 6 – 12 reps/side

FREQUENCY: 2 – 3 times per week

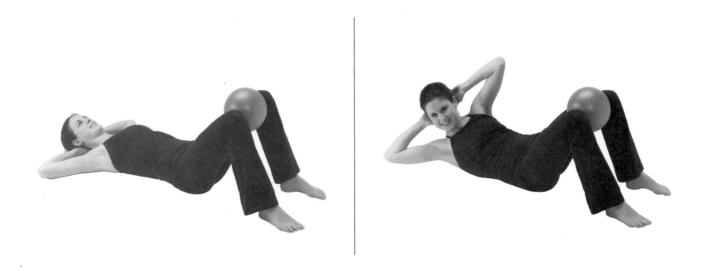

Instructions:
Lie on back with knees bent and ball between knees. Place unclasped hands behind head and gently draw lower abdomen toward spine. Gently squeeze shoulder blades together as you raise left elbow across body while keeping right elbow back. Press knees lightly into ball. Repeat on opposite side.

Pelvic Floor Strengthener

Level of Difficulty: ★☆☆☆☆

Benefits: Strengthens pelvic floor muscles.

HOLD: 3 – 20 seconds

REST: Twice as long as hold time

REPEAT: 3 – 10 repetitions

FREQUENCY: daily

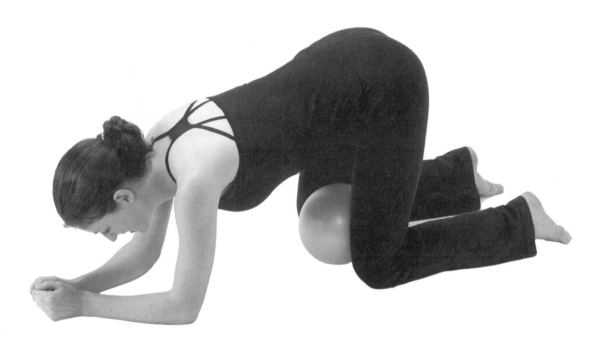

Instructions:
Kneel. Place ball between knees. Lean forward and place forearms on floor. Take a relaxed breath in and out. Now without breathing in, slowly draw the pelvic floor muscles up and in as if you are attempting to stop urine flow. Hold and breathe lightly.

Hip Twister

Level of Difficulty: ★ ★ ★ ☆ ☆

Benefits: Strengthens abdomen, arms, and hips.

REPEAT: 20 – 60 seconds

FREQUENCY: daily

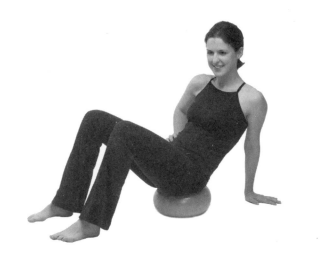 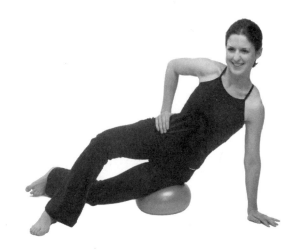

Instructions:

Sit on ball. Place right hand on hip. Lean back and place left hand flat on floor. Shift weight onto left hip as left bent leg moves under right knee. Return to starting position. Repeat with opposite side.

Thigh Squeeze

Level of Difficulty: ★☆☆☆☆

Benefits: Strengthens inner thigh and pelvic floor muscles.

HOLD: 3 seconds

REPEAT: 1 – 3 sets, 8 – 12 reps/side

FREQUENCY: 3 – 4 times per week

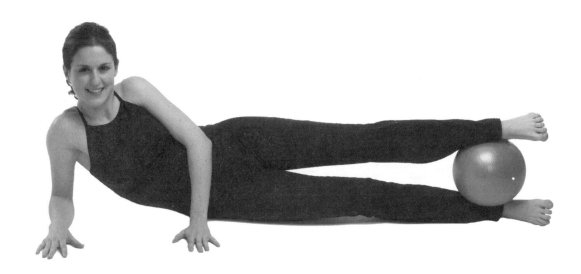

Instructions:
Lie on side with ball between ankles. Straighten legs, maintaining a straight line between ankle, hips, and shoulders. Draw lower abdomen toward spine. Squeeze ankles together. Repeat with opposite side.

Variation:
Perform as above, however after squeezing ankles together raise ankles off floor. Hold: 1 second; Repeat: 1 – 3 sets, 3 – 8 reps per side.

Level of Difficulty: ★ ★ ★ ★☆

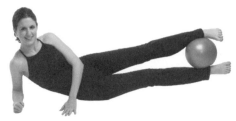

Hip Stabilizer

Level of Difficulty: ★☆☆☆☆

Benefits: Strengthens inner thigh and outer (gluteus medius) hip muscles.

HOLD: 3 seconds each direction

REPEAT: 1 – 3 sets, 8 – 12 reps / side

FREQUENCY: 3 – 4 times per week

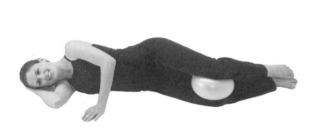 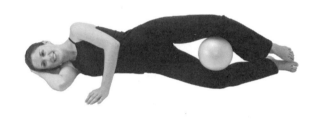

Instructions:
Lie on side with knees bent and feet aligned with trunk. Squeeze ball between knees. Hold. Gently release. Keeping heels together raise top knee up as far as possible without ball slipping. Repeat with opposite side.

Bicycle

Level of Difficulty: ★ ★ ★ ☆

Benefits: Strengthens abdominal and leg muscles.

REPEAT: 1 – 3 sets, 6 – 12 reps

FREQUENCY: 2 – 3 times per week

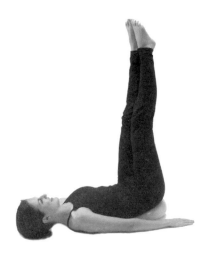
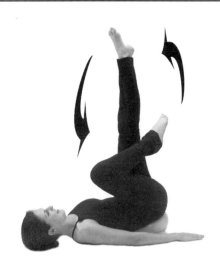

Instructions:
Lie on back with knees bent. Place ball beneath sacrum (pelvis). Gently draw lower abdomen toward spine and raise both feet off floor, one bent knee at a time. Slowly straighten legs and point toes. Move legs in a bicycle motion. Bend knees and return to starting position.

Alternate position:
Follow directions as above, however after straightening legs and pointing toes– move legs apart (into 'v' position) and back together. Repeat. This position will strengthen abdominal and inner thigh muscles. Hold: 3 seconds; Repeat: 1 – 3 sets, 6 – 12 reps per side; Frequency: 2 – 3 times per week.

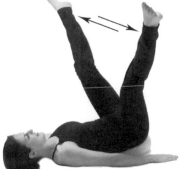

Level of Difficulty: ★ ★ ★ ☆

Pilates Leg Raises

Level of Difficulty: ★ ★ ★ ☆ ☆

Benefits: Strengthens abdominal, arm, and leg muscles.

HOLD: 3 seconds

REPEAT: 1 – 3 sets, 3 – 8 reps / side

FREQUENCY: 2 – 3 times per week

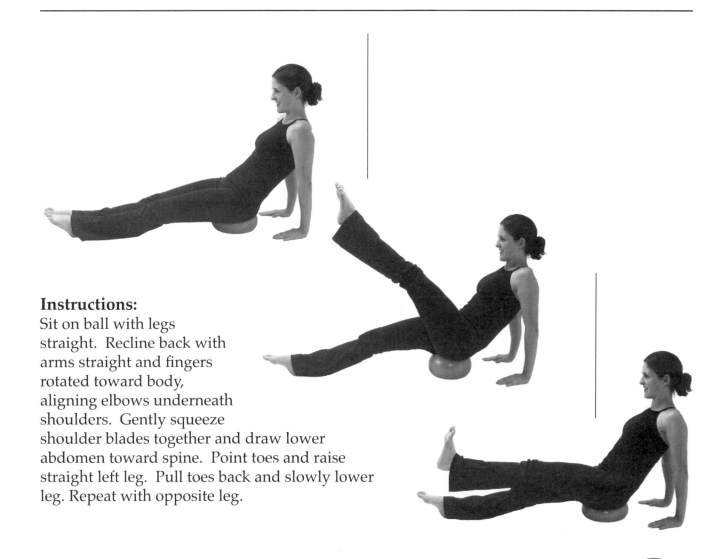

Instructions:
Sit on ball with legs straight. Recline back with arms straight and fingers rotated toward body, aligning elbows underneath shoulders. Gently squeeze shoulder blades together and draw lower abdomen toward spine. Point toes and raise straight left leg. Pull toes back and slowly lower leg. Repeat with opposite leg.

Straight Leg Raises

Level of Difficulty: ★★☆☆☆

Benefits: Strengthens inner thigh and pelvic floor muscles.

HOLD: 3 seconds	
REPEAT: 1 – 3 sets, 8 – 12 reps / side	
FREQUENCY: 3 – 4 times per week	

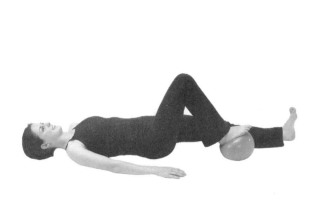
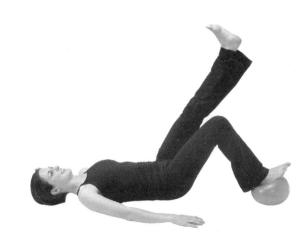

Instructions:
Lie on back with knees bent and ball positioned under foot. Gently draw lower abdomen toward spine. Straighten opposite leg and raise, with toes flexed, off floor.

Leg Circle Variation:
Perform exercise as above, however point toes and raise leg. Make small circles with foot. Reverse directions of circles. Repeat with opposite side.

Level of Difficulty: ★★★☆☆

37

Standing Heel Slides on Wall

Level of Difficulty: ★★☆☆☆

Benefits: Strengthens knee and thigh muscles.

HOLD: 3 seconds at end positions

REPEAT: 1 – 3 sets, 8 – 12 reps / side

FREQUENCY: 3 – 4 times per week

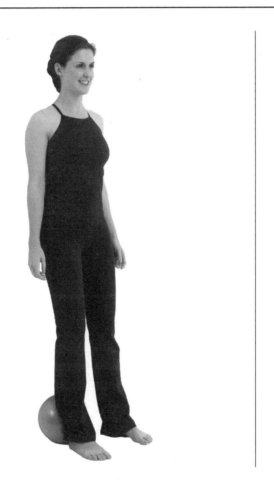
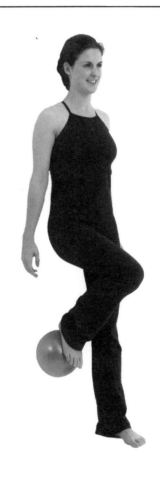

Instructions:
Stand with feet hip-width apart and back against wall. Bend knee and place ball behind heel. Gently draw lower abdomen toward spine. Straighten knee, keeping knee aligned over toes. Repeat on opposite side.

38

Mini-Squat with Ball Between Knees

Level of Difficulty: ★★★☆☆

Benefits: Strengthens legs, vastus medialis obliques (front thigh muscles), and buttock muscles.

HOLD: 3 seconds

REPEAT: 1 – 3 sets, 8 – 12 repetitions

FREQUENCY: 3 – 4 times per week

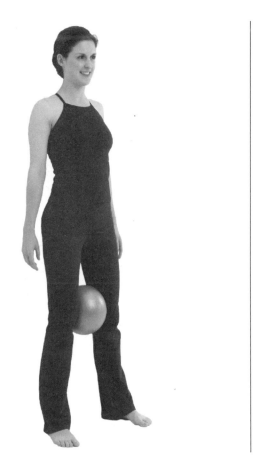
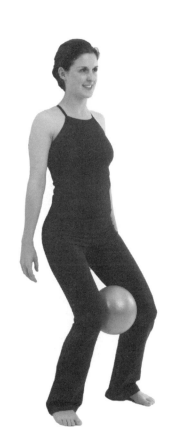

Instructions:
Stand with back against wall and place ball between knees. Gently draw lower abdomen toward spine. Perform a mini-squat to position of comfort, keeping knees aligned over toes. Return to standing position.

Mini-Squat with Shoulder Press Into Wall

Level of Difficulty: ★ ★ ★ ☆

Benefits: Strengthens arms, shoulders, abdomen, back, buttock, and leg muscles.

HOLD: 3 seconds

REPEAT: 1 – 3 sets, 8 – 12 repetitions

FREQUENCY: 3 – 4 times per week

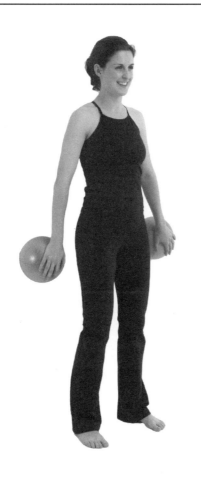
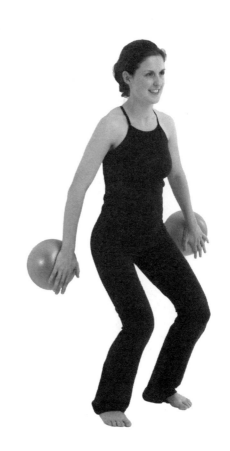

Instructions:
Stand with feet hip-width apart and back against wall. Grasp one ball in each hand. Gently draw lower abdomen toward spine. Perform a mini-squat keeping knees aligned over toes. Lightly press each palm into balls. Return to standing position.

40

Mini-Squat with Shoulder Protraction/Retraction

Level of Difficulty: ★ ★ ★ ★ ☆

Benefits: Strengthens mid back, chest, abdomen, back, buttock and leg muscles.

HOLD: 3 seconds

REPEAT: 1 – 3 sets, 8 – 12 reps / side

FREQUENCY: 3 – 4 times per week

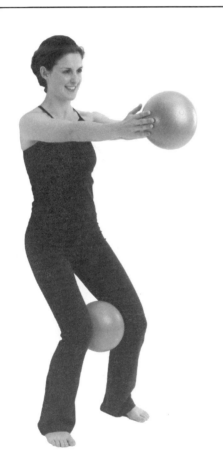
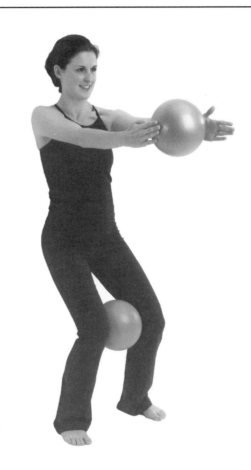

Instructions:
Stand with feet hip-width apart and back against wall. Place ball between palms. Gently draw lower abdomen toward spine. Perform a mini-squat keeping knees aligned over toes. Lightly press palms into ball. Raise straight arms to 90 degrees. Slowly slide right hand away from body and left hand toward body. Repeat in opposite direction.

Mini-Squat with Tricep Extension

Level of Difficulty: ★ ★ ★ ★ ☆

Benefits: Strengthens back of arms (triceps), abdomen, back, legs, thighs, and buttocks.

HOLD: 3 seconds

REPEAT: 1 – 3 sets, 8 – 12 repetitions

FREQUENCY: 3 – 4 times per week

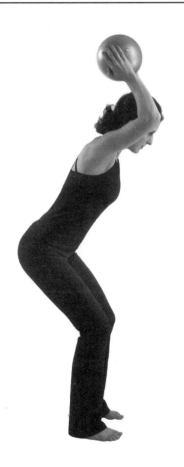 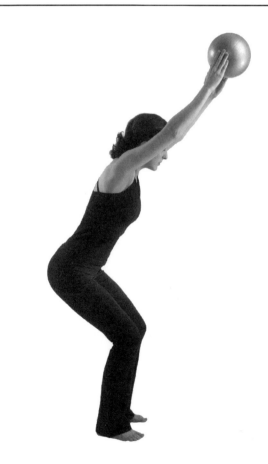

Instructions:
Stand with feet hip-width apart and place ball between palms. Gently draw lower abdomen toward spine. Perform a mini-squat keeping knees aligned over toes. Raise arms so they align with spine. Bend elbows and lower ball behind back. Straighten arms. Return to starting position.

42

Mini-Squat with Arm Raises

Level of Difficulty: ★ ★ ★ ★ ☆

Benefits: Strengthens arms, abdomen, back, buttock, and leg muscles.

HOLD: 3 seconds

REPEAT: 1 – 3 sets, 8 – 12 repetitions

FREQUENCY: 3 – 4 times per week

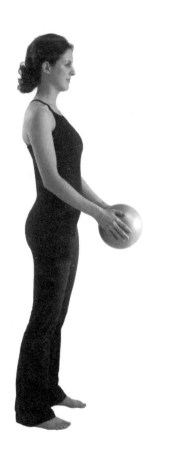
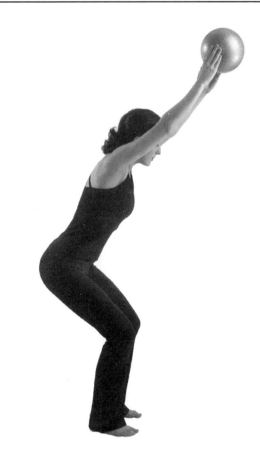

Instructions:
Stand with feet hip-width apart and grasp one ball in each hand. Gently draw lower abdomen toward spine. Perform a mini-squat, keeping knees aligned over toes, and raise arms so they align with spine. Lightly press each palm into balls. Return to standing position.

43

Modified Cactus Pose

Level of Difficulty: ★★★★☆

Benefits: Strengthens thighs, legs, buttocks, and mid-back areas.

HOLD: 3 seconds

REPEAT: 1 – 3 sets, 3 – 6 reps/side

FREQUENCY: 3 – 4 times per week

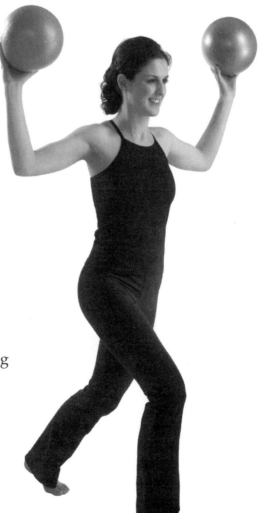

Instructions:
Stand with feet hip-width apart and grasp one ball in each hand. Gently draw lower abdomen toward spine. Lunge forward with one foot forward, keeping knee aligned over foot, and one foot back, raising back heel off floor while raising arms overhead. Bend elbows to 90 degrees and draw shoulder blades down and in. Hold. Return to standing position. Repeat on opposite side.

References

Craig, Colleen. 2003. *Abs on the Ball: A Pilates Approach to Building Superb Abdominals.*
 Rochester, VT: Inner Traditions International, LTD.

Creager, C.C. 2001. *Bounce Back Into Shape After Baby.* Berthoud, CO: FitNiche
 Publications.

Creager, C. C. 2006. *Core Strength Training Using Inflatable and Foam Rollers.*
 Berthoud, CO: FitNiche Publishing.

Creager, C.C. 2001. "Foam Rollers Facilitate Core Stability." *WorldWideSpine &
 Industrial Rehabilitation* 1(1): 16-19.

Creager C.C. 1996. *Therapeutic Exercises Using Foam Rollers.* Berthoud, CO:
 Executive Physical Therapy.

Creager, C.C. 1994. *Therapeutic Exercises Using the Swiss Ball.* Berthoud, CO:
 Executive Physical Therapy.

Lee, Diane. 2004. *The Pelvic Girdle: An approach to the examination and treatment of
 the lumbopelvic-hip region.* London: Churchill Livingstone.

Richardson, C., Jull, G., Hodges, P., and Hides, J. 2004. *Therapeutic
 Exercise for Lumbopelvic Stabilization.* London: Churchill Livingstone.

Sahrmann, S.A. 2002. *Diagnosis and Treatment of Movement Impairment Syndromes.*
 St. Louis, MO: Mosby.

SoftGym with the Overball and other Gymnic Softballs. Osoppo, Italy.
 Ledraplastic Spa.